# Empower Your Essence: A Holistic Guide to Health and Vitality

## Discover the Secrets to Nourishing Your Mind, Body, and Soul

# Chapters

# 14. Balancing Taste, Fuel, and Enjoyment

Introduction:
This book is for anyone seeking to embark on a journey of holistic well-being, nourishing their mind, body, and soul to unlock their full potential and live a life filled with vitality and joy. In today's fast-paced world, it's easy to neglect our holistic health in favor of quick fixes and temporary solutions. However, true vitality comes from nurturing all aspects of our being – physical, mental, and emotional. Through the insights and practices shared in this book, readers will gain a deeper understanding of their bodies and minds, empowering them to make informed choices that support their overall well-being. Whether you're looking to improve your physical fitness, enhance mental clarity, or cultivate emotional resilience, this book provides the tools and guidance you need to embark on a transformative journey of self-discovery and empowerment.

# Chapter 1: Unveiling the Essence of Holistic Well-being

*Proverbial Insight:*
"Healthy mind, healthy body." As we embark on our journey to holistic well-being, let's unveil the essence of what it truly means to live a balanced and fulfilling life.

In today's fast-paced world, it's easy to get caught up in the hustle and bustle of daily life. But amidst the chaos, lies the opportunity to reconnect with ourselves and embrace the holistic essence of well-being. This chapter serves as a guide to uncovering the foundational principles that shape our physical, mental, and emotional health.

Rediscovering Movement Patterns: Think about the simple acts of bending down to tie your shoes, reaching for something on a high shelf, or walking up a flight of stairs. These are all examples of basic movement patterns that we perform every day without even realizing it. By understanding and mastering these patterns – such as squatting, bending, pushing, pulling, twisting, walking, and lunging – we can enhance our mobility, strength, and overall functionality. For instance, practicing squats not only strengthens our leg muscles but also improves our ability to perform daily tasks like getting in and out of chairs or picking up objects from the ground.

Proverbial Reflection:
"Practice makes perfect." Just like mastering a new skill takes time and dedication, so does mastering our movement patterns. Consistent practice and gradual progression are key to unlocking our body's full potential.

Exploring Mindful Movement:
Incorporating movement into our daily lives doesn't have to mean hitting the gym for an intense workout. It can be as simple as taking a brisk walk during your lunch break, stretching while watching TV, or playing with your kids at the park. By infusing mindfulness into our movements, we become more present in the moment and cultivate a deeper connection with our bodies.

Proverbial Wisdom:
"Listen to your body." Pay attention to how your body feels during different movements. If something doesn't feel right, adjust your technique or try a different approach. Your body knows best.

Understanding the Mind-Body Connection:
Our physical health is intricately linked to our mental and emotional

well-being. When we move our bodies, we release endorphins – feel-good hormones that can boost our mood and reduce stress. Similarly, when we engage in activities that nourish our minds, such as meditation or journaling, we create a sense of inner peace and harmony that positively impacts our overall health.

Proverbial Reflection:
"Healthy habits, healthy mind." Cultivating healthy habits, both physically and mentally, contributes to a balanced and resilient mind-body connection. Consider incorporating activities like yoga, meditation, or deep breathing exercises into your daily routine to promote holistic well-being.

Practical Application:
To incorporate the principles of holistic movement into your daily life,

start by identifying areas where you can add more activity. Take the stairs instead of the elevator, go for a walk with a friend instead of meeting for coffee, or try a new exercise class that piques your interest. Remember, it's not about perfection; it's about progress. By taking small steps each day, you can gradually build a foundation of holistic well-being that supports you in living your best life.

## Chapter 2: The Science of Nourishing Your Body

*Proverbial Insight:*
"You are what you eat." As we dive into the science of nutrition, let's explore how the foods we choose impact our bodies and overall well-being.

Nutrition is the cornerstone of health, yet navigating the world of food choices can feel overwhelming at times. In this chapter, we'll unpack the science behind nourishing your body and discover practical ways to make informed dietary decisions.

Understanding Nutrient Chemistry: Imagine your body as a complex machine, with each nutrient playing a unique role in keeping it running smoothly. Carbohydrates, for example, are like the fuel that powers your engine, providing the energy needed for daily activities. Proteins act as the building blocks, repairing and maintaining tissues, while fats serve as the lubricant, ensuring everything operates smoothly. By understanding the chemistry of nutrients, we can make smarter choices about the foods we consume.

Practical Application:
Next time you're planning a meal,

think about incorporating a balance of carbohydrates, proteins, and fats. For example, a meal of grilled chicken (protein), brown rice (carbohydrates), and avocado (healthy fats) provides a well-rounded combination of nutrients to fuel your body and keep you satisfied.

Exploring Micronutrients:
In addition to macronutrients like carbohydrates, proteins, and fats, our bodies also require a variety of micronutrients – vitamins and minerals – to function optimally. These micronutrients act as co-factors in biochemical reactions, supporting everything from energy production to immune function. For example, vitamin C is essential for collagen synthesis and immune health, while calcium is crucial for bone strength and muscle function.

Proverbial Wisdom:
"An apple a day keeps the doctor away." While it may sound cliché, there's truth to the adage that whole, nutrient-dense foods are key to maintaining health and vitality. Incorporating a variety of fruits, vegetables, lean proteins, and whole grains into your diet ensures you're getting a diverse array of micronutrients to support your body's needs.

Navigating Modern Food Choices:
In today's fast-paced world, convenience often trumps nutrition when it comes to food choices. Processed and convenience foods may be convenient, but they're often lacking in essential nutrients and loaded with unhealthy additives. By prioritizing whole, minimally processed foods, we can nourish our bodies with the nutrients they need to thrive.

Practical Application:
When grocery shopping, focus on filling your cart with whole foods like fruits, vegetables, lean proteins, and whole grains. Opt for fresh or frozen produce over canned varieties, and choose products with minimal added sugars, preservatives, and artificial ingredients.

Incorporating the science of nutrition into your daily life doesn't have to be complicated. By understanding the role of macronutrients and micronutrients and making informed food choices, you can nourish your body from the inside out and support your overall health and well-being. Remember, small changes can lead to big results, so start by incorporating one healthy choice at a time and watch as your body thrives.

# Chapter 3: Embracing Intermittent Fasting

*Proverbial Insight:*
"A break from food is a break for the body." As we delve into the realm of intermittent fasting, let's explore how this eating pattern can benefit our bodies and support overall health.

Intermittent fasting has gained popularity in recent years as a flexible and effective approach to managing weight and promoting wellness. In this chapter, we'll uncover the principles of intermittent fasting and discover practical ways to incorporate it into our everyday lives.

Understanding Intermittent Fasting: Intermittent fasting involves alternating periods of eating and fasting, rather than focusing solely on what foods to eat. This approach taps into our body's natural rhythm, allowing for periods of rest and repair between meals. There are several different methods of intermittent fasting, including the 16/8 method, where you fast for 16 hours and eat during an 8-hour window, and the 5:2 method, where you eat normally for five days and restrict calories for two non-consecutive days.

Practical Application:
One way to ease into intermittent fasting is to start with a shorter fasting window, such as 12 hours overnight. For example, if you finish dinner at 7 p.m., you would wait until 7 a.m. the next day before eating breakfast. As you become more comfortable with fasting, you can gradually extend the fasting window to suit your preferences and lifestyle.

Benefits of Intermittent Fasting:
Intermittent fasting offers more than just weight loss benefits; it can also improve metabolic health, increase energy levels, and support cellular repair processes. By giving our bodies a break from constant digestion, we allow them to focus on other important functions, such as detoxification and repair. Additionally, intermittent fasting has been shown to reduce inflammation, improve insulin sensitivity, and enhance brain function.

Practical Application:
To reap the benefits of intermittent fasting, focus on eating nutrient-dense meals during your eating window and staying hydrated throughout the day. Experiment with different fasting protocols to find what works best for your body and lifestyle, and listen to your body's hunger and satiety cues.

Proverbial Wisdom:
"Patience is bitter, but its fruit is sweet." While intermittent fasting may require an adjustment period, the long-term benefits are well worth the effort. Trust the process and be patient with yourself as you explore this eating pattern.

Intermittent fasting offers a flexible and sustainable approach to promoting health and well-being. By embracing this eating pattern and incorporating it into our daily lives, we can unlock a multitude of benefits for our bodies and minds. Remember, intermittent fasting is not about deprivation or restriction; it's about giving our bodies the time and space they need to thrive. So, embrace the rhythm of intermittent fasting and discover the transformative power it can have on your overall health and vitality.

## Chapter 4: Finding Balance with Portion Control and Food Harmony

*Proverbial Insight:*
"A portion in hand is worth two on the plate." As we explore the art of portion control and food harmony, let's uncover how these practices can support a balanced and satisfying approach to eating.

In today's world of supersized meals and endless food options, finding balance when it comes to portion sizes and food combinations can be challenging. In this chapter, we'll delve into the importance of portion control and creating harmonious meals that nourish both body and soul.

Understanding Portion Control:
Portion control is about more than

just limiting the amount of food we eat; it's also about being mindful of how much we need to feel satisfied. One practical way to practice portion control is to use visual cues, such as comparing serving sizes to everyday objects like a deck of cards or a tennis ball. Additionally, paying attention to hunger and fullness cues can help us avoid overeating and better tune in to our body's natural signals.

Practical Application:
When serving yourself a meal, start by filling half your plate with vegetables, a quarter with lean protein, and a quarter with whole grains or starchy vegetables. This balanced approach ensures you're getting a variety of nutrients while also keeping portion sizes in check.

Creating Food Harmony:
Food harmony is about finding the

perfect balance of flavors, textures, and nutrients to create meals that not only satisfy our hunger but also nourish our bodies and souls. One way to achieve food harmony is to focus on creating balanced meals that include a variety of colors, flavors, and food groups. For example, pairing sweet potatoes with black beans and avocado creates a harmonious blend of carbohydrates, protein, and healthy fats.

Practical Application:
Experiment with different flavor combinations and cooking techniques to create meals that excite your taste buds and satisfy your hunger. Try incorporating fresh herbs, spices, and citrus zest to add depth and complexity to your dishes, and don't be afraid to get creative with your ingredient choices.

Proverbial Wisdom:
"Variety is the spice of life." Embrace the diversity of foods available to you and experiment with different combinations to keep meals interesting and enjoyable.
Remember, there's no one-size-fits-all approach to portion control and food harmony; it's about finding what works best for you and your body.

By practicing portion control and creating food harmony in our meals, we can cultivate a balanced and satisfying approach to eating that supports our overall health and well-being. Remember, it's not about deprivation or restriction; it's about finding joy and satisfaction in every bite. So, embrace the art of portion control and food harmony, and discover the transformative power they can have on your relationship with food and your quality of life.

## Chapter 5: Smart Strategies for Starches and Energy

*Proverbial Insight:*
"Starch wisely, live energetically." As we delve into the world of starches and their impact on energy levels, let's uncover practical strategies for making smart carbohydrate choices that support our overall well-being.

Starches often get a bad rap in the world of nutrition, but they play a vital role in providing our bodies with the energy they need to function optimally. In this chapter, we'll explore how to navigate the world of starches strategically to maintain steady energy levels throughout the day.

Understanding Starches:
Starches are complex carbohydrates found in foods like grains, legumes, and starchy vegetables. While they're

an important source of energy, not all starches are created equal. Refined starches, like white bread and pastries, can cause spikes and crashes in blood sugar levels, leading to feelings of fatigue and sluggishness. On the other hand, whole grains, beans, and root vegetables provide a steady source of energy thanks to their fiber content and slower digestion rate.

Practical Application:
Swap out refined starches for whole grain alternatives like brown rice, quinoa, or whole wheat pasta. These options provide more fiber and nutrients, helping to keep you feeling satisfied and energized for longer periods.

Strategic Choices for Energy:
When it comes to fueling our bodies for energy, timing and portion size are key. Instead of loading up on

starches all at once, aim to spread your carbohydrate intake evenly throughout the day to maintain steady blood sugar levels and avoid energy crashes. Pairing starches with protein and healthy fats can also help slow digestion and provide a more sustained release of energy.

Practical Application:
Start your day with a balanced breakfast that includes a mix of carbohydrates, protein, and healthy fats, such as oatmeal topped with nuts and fruit or whole grain toast with avocado and eggs. This combination sets the stage for stable energy levels and sustained focus throughout the morning.

Proverbial Wisdom:
"Slow and steady wins the race." By choosing whole, nutrient-dense starches and spreading our carbohydrate intake evenly

throughout the day, we can maintain steady energy levels and avoid the highs and lows associated with refined starches.

Starches are an important part of a balanced diet, providing our bodies with the energy they need to thrive. By making smart choices and incorporating whole, nutrient-dense options into our meals, we can fuel our bodies for optimal performance and enjoy sustained energy throughout the day. So, starch wisely and live energetically, knowing that the choices you make can have a profound impact on your overall well-being and vitality.

## Chapter 6: Mastering Movement for Everyday Empowerment

*Proverbial Insight:*
"Move it or lose it." As we embark on

a journey to master movement patterns, let's explore how everyday movements can empower us to live our best lives.

Movement is more than just exercise; it's a fundamental aspect of being human. In this chapter, we'll uncover the power of mastering movement patterns and how they can enhance our everyday lives.

Exploring Everyday Movement:
Think about the simple actions you perform every day, from sitting and standing to bending and reaching. These movements are the building blocks of functional fitness and play a crucial role in maintaining mobility, strength, and independence as we age. By mastering these basic movement patterns – such as squatting, bending, pushing, pulling, twisting, walking, and lunging – we

can improve our quality of life and reduce the risk of injury.

Practical Application:
Incorporate movement into your daily routine by taking the stairs instead of the elevator, squatting to pick up objects from the ground, or practicing balance exercises while brushing your teeth. These simple actions not only strengthen your muscles but also improve your mobility and coordination.

Empowering Mind-Body Connection:
Our bodies are designed to move, and every movement we make sends signals to our brain that enhance our overall well-being. By embracing a variety of movement patterns, we can improve our balance, coordination, and proprioception – the body's awareness of its position in space. This heightened mind-body connection not only improves

physical performance but also enhances mental clarity and focus.

Practical Application:
Engage in activities that challenge your coordination and balance, such as yoga, tai chi, or dancing. These practices not only improve physical function but also cultivate mindfulness and presence in everyday life.

Proverbial Wisdom:
"Use it or lose it." Regular movement is essential for maintaining mobility and function throughout life. By incorporating a variety of movements into our daily lives, we can empower ourselves to live with vitality and independence.

Mastering movement patterns is not just about exercise; it's about embracing a lifestyle of empowerment and vitality. By prioritizing everyday movements and incorporating them into our daily routines, we can enhance our physical and mental well-being and live our best lives. So, move with purpose and intention, knowing that every step you take brings you closer to a life filled with strength, resilience, and joy.

## Chapter 7: Unleashing Your Strength, Range, and Mobility

*Proverbial Insight:*
"Strength begins with a single step." As we dive into the exploration of our physical capabilities, let's uncover how understanding our strength, range, and mobility can empower us in our daily lives.

Our bodies are capable of incredible feats, from lifting heavy objects to reaching for distant heights. In this chapter, we'll explore how unlocking our strength, range, and mobility can enhance our overall well-being and empower us to tackle life's challenges with confidence.

Discovering Your Strength:
Strength is not just about how much weight you can lift; it's about having the physical capacity to perform daily tasks with ease and confidence. By engaging in strength-building exercises, such as squats, lunges, and push-ups, we can improve our muscle mass, bone density, and overall functional capacity. Strength training also boosts metabolism, enhances posture, and reduces the risk of injury.

Practical Application:
Incorporate bodyweight exercises into your daily routine, such as wall sits while brushing your teeth, or lunges while waiting for the kettle to boil. These simple movements

strengthen your muscles and improve your functional capacity without the need for equipment.

Exploring Range of Motion:
Range of motion refers to the extent to which we can move our joints through their full range of motion. Maintaining good flexibility and mobility is essential for preventing injury, reducing muscle tension, and improving overall movement efficiency. By incorporating stretching and mobility exercises into our daily routine, we can enhance our range of motion and move more freely.

Practical Application:
Start and end your day with a few minutes of stretching to improve flexibility and mobility. Focus on areas of tightness or discomfort, such as the hips, shoulders, and spine, and perform gentle stretches

to release tension and improve range of motion.

Empowering Mobility:
Mobility is the ability to move freely and easily without restriction or pain. It encompasses not only flexibility but also stability, coordination, and balance. By incorporating dynamic movements and balance exercises into our daily routine, we can improve our mobility and reduce the risk of falls and injuries as we age.

Practical Application:
Practice balance exercises like standing on one leg while brushing your teeth or walking heel-to-toe along a straight line. These activities challenge your stability and coordination and improve overall mobility and balance.

Proverbial Wisdom:
"Strength is not measured by what you can lift, but by what you can

carry." By understanding and embracing our strength, range, and mobility, we can navigate life's challenges with confidence and grace.

Unleashing our strength, range, and mobility is not just about physical prowess; it's about reclaiming our inherent capability to move with ease and confidence. By prioritizing strength training, flexibility, and mobility exercises in our daily lives, we can enhance our physical well-being and empower ourselves to live life to the fullest. So, embrace your strength, expand your range, and unleash your mobility, knowing that the power to live a vibrant and fulfilling life lies within you.

## Chapter 8: Daily Habits for Empowered Fitness

*Proverbial Insight:*
"Small steps lead to big gains." As we delve into the realm of daily fitness rituals, let's uncover how establishing empowering habits can transform our lives one step at a time.

*Introduction:*
Fitness is not just about hitting the gym; it's about cultivating daily habits that support our physical and mental well-being. In this chapter, we'll explore simple yet powerful daily rituals that can empower us to lead healthier, more active lives.

Morning Movement:
Starting your day with movement sets a positive tone for the hours ahead. Whether it's a quick yoga flow, a brisk walk, or a few minutes of stretching, incorporating morning movement into your routine wakes up your body and mind, boosts

energy levels, and improves mood and focus for the day ahead.

Practical Application:
Set aside just 10 minutes each morning for a mini workout routine. This could include bodyweight exercises like squats, lunges, and push-ups, or simple stretches to wake up your muscles and joints.

Midday Movement Breaks:
Sitting for prolonged periods can take a toll on our bodies and minds. Incorporating short movement breaks throughout the day can counteract the negative effects of sedentary behavior, improve circulation, and alleviate stiffness and tension. Take a quick walk around the office, stretch at your desk, or do a few simple exercises to keep your body moving and your mind engaged.

Practical Application:
Set a timer to remind yourself to take a movement break every hour. Stand up, stretch your arms overhead, roll your shoulders, and take a few deep breaths to refresh your body and mind.

Evening Wind-Down:
As the day winds down, it's important to prioritize relaxation and recovery to prepare for restorative sleep. Engaging in calming activities like gentle yoga, meditation, or foam rolling can help release tension, reduce stress, and promote deep relaxation for a restful night's sleep.

Practical Application:
Create a bedtime routine that includes relaxation practices like gentle stretching, deep breathing exercises, or a warm bath. Establishing a calming bedtime ritual signals to your body that it's time to

unwind and prepares you for a restful night's sleep.

Proverbial Wisdom:
"Consistency is key." By incorporating daily fitness rituals into our lives, we lay the foundation for long-term health and well-being. Consistent effort, even in small doses, leads to significant progress over time.

Daily fitness rituals are the building blocks of a healthy, active lifestyle. By prioritizing movement throughout the day and establishing empowering habits that support our physical and mental well-being, we can unlock our full potential and thrive in every aspect of life. So, embrace the power of daily movement, one step at a time, knowing that each small action brings you closer to a life of vitality, resilience, and joy.

## Chapter 9: Vitality Through Respiration, Circulation, and Perspiration

*Proverbial Insight:*
"Breathe deeply, live fully." As we explore the pillars of holistic fitness, let's uncover how focusing on respiration, circulation, and perspiration can invigorate our bodies and elevate our vitality.

Our bodies are intricate systems that rely on essential processes like respiration, circulation, and perspiration to function optimally. In this chapter, we'll dive into the importance of these three pillars of holistic fitness and discover how they contribute to our overall well-being.

Harnessing the Power of Respiration: Breathing is one of the most fundamental and yet often overlooked aspects of health and vitality. Deep, diaphragmatic breathing not only oxygenates our cells but also calms the nervous system, reduces stress, and enhances mental clarity and focus. By practicing mindful breathing techniques like belly breathing or alternate nostril breathing, we can tap into the restorative power of our breath and support our physical and emotional well-being.

Practical Application:
Take a few moments throughout the day to pause and focus on your breath. Close your eyes, place one hand on your belly, and take slow, deep breaths, allowing your abdomen to rise and fall with each inhale and exhale. Notice how this simple practice helps you feel more grounded and centered in the present moment.

Optimizing Circulation:
Healthy circulation is essential for delivering oxygen and nutrients to our cells, removing waste products, and maintaining overall vitality. Regular physical activity, such as walking, cycling, or swimming, promotes circulation by increasing blood flow to the muscles and organs, strengthening the heart, and improving cardiovascular health. Additionally, practices like dry brushing or hydrotherapy can stimulate circulation and enhance detoxification, leaving you feeling rejuvenated and energized.

Practical Application:
Incorporate movement into your daily routine to promote circulation and vitality. Take a brisk walk around the neighborhood, dance to your favorite music, or do a few minutes of jumping jacks to get your blood

flowing and invigorate your body and mind.

Embracing Perspiration:
Perspiration, or sweating, is the body's natural mechanism for regulating temperature and eliminating toxins. Engaging in activities that induce sweat, such as exercise, sauna sessions, or hot yoga, not only helps cool the body but also supports detoxification, boosts metabolism, and enhances skin health. By embracing perspiration as a natural and beneficial process, we can unlock the full potential of our bodies and promote overall well-being.

Practical Application:
Schedule regular sweat sessions into your weekly routine to promote detoxification and vitality. Whether it's hitting the gym, taking a hot yoga class, or simply spending time

outdoors in warm weather, prioritize activities that induce sweat and leave you feeling refreshed and rejuvenated.

Proverbial Wisdom:
"Every breath is a gift, every heartbeat a miracle." By nurturing our respiration, circulation, and perspiration, we honor the incredible gift of life and empower ourselves to live with vitality and purpose.

Respiration, circulation, and perspiration are not just physiological processes; they are the foundation of holistic fitness and vitality. By prioritizing practices that support these essential functions – from mindful breathing to regular exercise to embracing sweat – we can cultivate a deep sense of well-being and thrive in every aspect of life. So, breathe deeply, move freely, and sweat often, knowing that by nurturing these pillars of health, you are nurturing the essence of your vitality and vitality.

## Chapter 10: Mindful Cardiovascular Engagement

*Proverbial Insight:*
"A strong heart beats in rhythm with life." As we embark on a journey of cardiovascular engagement, let's explore how mindful approaches to heart-pumping activities can not only improve fitness but also enhance mental well-being.

*Introduction:*
Cardiovascular exercise is often associated with physical fitness, but its benefits extend far beyond the body. In this chapter, we'll delve into the joy of heart-pumping activities and discover how they can elevate

not only our fitness levels but also our mental and emotional well-being.

Exploring Heart-Pumping Activities: Cardiovascular exercises, such as running, cycling, or dancing, get our hearts pumping and our blood flowing, providing a myriad of benefits for our bodies and minds. Engaging in these activities not only improves cardiovascular health by strengthening the heart and lungs but also boosts mood, reduces stress, and enhances cognitive function. By approaching cardiovascular exercise with mindfulness and intention, we can maximize its benefits and cultivate a deeper connection with our bodies.

Practical Application:
Choose activities that you enjoy and that align with your fitness goals. Whether it's going for a jog in nature, attending a dance class with friends,

or cycling through your neighborhood, find ways to incorporate heart-pumping activities into your routine that bring you joy and fulfillment.

Mindful Movement for Mental Well-Being:
Cardiovascular exercise has been shown to release endorphins, neurotransmitters that promote feelings of happiness and euphoria, and reduce levels of stress hormones like cortisol. Additionally, engaging in rhythmic activities, such as running or dancing, can induce a meditative state of flow, where you become fully immersed in the present moment and experience a sense of calm and clarity. By approaching cardiovascular exercise as a form of moving meditation, we can tap into its transformative power to improve mental well-being and enhance overall quality of life.

Practical Application:
Practice mindfulness during your cardiovascular workouts by focusing on your breath, tuning into the rhythm of your movements, and letting go of distractions and worries. Notice how this mindful approach enhances your enjoyment of the activity and leaves you feeling energized and uplifted.

Proverbial Wisdom:
"A healthy heart is a happy heart." By engaging in heart-pumping activities with mindfulness and intention, we not only strengthen our bodies but also nourish our souls, cultivating a deep sense of joy and vitality.

Mindful cardiovascular engagement offers a pathway to improved fitness, mental well-being, and overall vitality. By approaching heart-pumping activities with mindfulness and intention, we can unlock their transformative power to enhance our physical, mental, and emotional health. So, lace up your sneakers, tune into the rhythm of your heart, and embrace the joy of movement, knowing that each step brings you closer to a life filled with strength, happiness, and vitality.

## Chapter 11: Unveiling the Strength Within

*Proverbial Insight:*
"Strength is not just physical; it's also mental and emotional." As we explore the importance of strength training, let's uncover how it contributes to our overall health and vitality.

Strength training is more than just lifting weights; it's about cultivating resilience and empowerment from the inside out. In this chapter, we'll delve into the transformative power of strength training and discover how it can enhance our physical, mental, and emotional well-being.

Discovering the Essence of Strength:
Strength is not solely about muscle size or physical prowess; it's about tapping into our inner resilience and harnessing our innate power to overcome obstacles. Strength training builds not only physical strength but also mental and emotional fortitude, teaching us to push past our limits, embrace challenges, and cultivate a mindset of resilience and perseverance.

Practical Application:
Incorporate strength training exercises into your routine that challenge both your body and mind. This could include bodyweight exercises like push-ups, squats, and planks, or resistance training with dumbbells, resistance bands, or

kettlebells. Focus on proper form and technique, and gradually increase the intensity and resistance as you progress.

Strength Beyond the Gym:
The benefits of strength training extend far beyond the gym. Building physical strength enhances our ability to perform daily tasks with ease and confidence, reduces the risk of injury, and improves overall functional capacity. Additionally, strength training boosts metabolism, enhances bone density, and promotes healthy aging, allowing us to live with vitality and independence as we age.

Practical Application:
Think about the activities you engage in throughout the day that require physical strength, such as lifting groceries, carrying laundry, or playing with children or grandchildren. By

incorporating strength training into your routine, you can improve your performance in these activities and enjoy a higher quality of life.

Proverbial Wisdom:
"Strength doesn't come from what you can do; it comes from overcoming the things you once thought you couldn't." By embracing strength training as a journey of self-discovery and empowerment, we unlock the limitless potential within us to overcome challenges and thrive in every aspect of life.

Strength training is not just about building muscle; it's about building resilience, empowerment, and vitality from the inside out. By incorporating strength training into our lives, we strengthen not only our bodies but also our minds and spirits, empowering ourselves to face life's challenges with confidence and grace. So, embrace the strength within you, knowing that with each lift, you are one step closer to unlocking your full potential and living a life of strength, resilience, and vitality.

## Chapter 12: The Power of Sweat: Detoxify and Energize

*Proverbial Insight:*
"Sweat cleanses the body and invigorates the soul." As we delve into the significance of perspiration, let's uncover how intentional sweating can rejuvenate our bodies and enhance our vitality.

Sweating is more than just a response to physical exertion; it's a natural detoxification process that cleanses our bodies from the inside out. In this chapter, we'll explore the transformative power of sweat and discover how incorporating intentional sweating into our lives can promote detoxification and energize our bodies.

Understanding the Role of Perspiration:
Perspiration, or sweating, is the body's way of regulating temperature and eliminating toxins. When we sweat, our pores open up, releasing built-up toxins, heavy metals, and metabolic waste from our bodies. By engaging in activities that induce sweat, such as exercise, sauna sessions, or hot yoga, we can support our body's natural detoxification processes and enhance overall health and vitality.

Practical Application:
Incorporate intentional sweating into your routine by engaging in activities that induce sweat and promote detoxification. This could include

high-intensity interval training (HIIT) workouts, hot yoga classes, or relaxing sauna sessions. Aim to sweat for at least 20-30 minutes several times a week to reap the benefits of detoxification and rejuvenation.

The Benefits of Detoxification: Detoxification not only cleanses our bodies of harmful toxins but also promotes overall well-being and vitality. By eliminating toxins and metabolic waste, detoxification supports healthy digestion, boosts immune function, and enhances skin health. Additionally, sweating has been shown to improve circulation, reduce inflammation, and promote relaxation, leaving us feeling refreshed, rejuvenated, and energized.

Practical Application:
Pay attention to how your body feels

after a good sweat session. Notice the increased energy, improved mood, and sense of well-being that accompanies detoxification. Use this as motivation to incorporate regular sweating into your routine and prioritize your body's natural cleansing processes.

Proverbial Wisdom:
"Sweat is the evidence of your hard work and dedication." By embracing intentional sweating as a form of self-care and rejuvenation, we honor our bodies' innate ability to cleanse and renew themselves, promoting overall health and vitality.

Intentional sweating is not just about physical exertion; it's about harnessing the transformative power of sweat to detoxify and energize our bodies from the inside out. By incorporating activities that induce sweat into our routine and prioritizing our body's natural cleansing processes, we can support overall health and well-being, and embrace a life filled with vitality and energy. So, embrace the power of sweat, knowing that with each drop, you are cleansing and revitalizing your body, mind, and soul.

## Chapter 13: The Chemistry of Nutrition: Nourish Your Body, Fuel Your Life

*Proverbial Insight:*
"Food is the fuel that powers our bodies and minds." As we explore the nourishing chemistry of food, let's uncover how making nutrient-dense choices can optimize our health and vitality.

Nutrition is more than just calories; it's about providing our bodies with the essential nutrients they need to thrive. In this chapter, we'll delve into the chemistry of food and discover how choosing nutrient-dense options can fuel our bodies and enrich our lives.

Understanding Nutrient Chemistry: Every bite we take is composed of various nutrients – vitamins, minerals, carbohydrates, proteins, and fats – each playing a crucial role in supporting our body's functions and promoting overall health. By understanding the chemistry of food and making informed choices, we can nourish our bodies at the cellular level and optimize our health and vitality.

Practical Application:
Focus on incorporating whole, nutrient-dense foods into your diet, such as fruits, vegetables, lean proteins, whole grains, and healthy fats. These foods provide a wealth of

essential nutrients, vitamins, and minerals that fuel your body and support optimal health.

Fueling Your Body's Optimal Function:
Food serves as the fuel that powers our bodies and minds, providing the energy and nutrients needed for daily activities, exercise, and cognitive function. By choosing nutrient-dense foods that provide sustained energy and support metabolic function, we can optimize our physical and mental performance and enhance overall well-being.

Practical Application:
Pay attention to how different foods make you feel and how they impact your energy levels and mood. Choose foods that provide sustained energy and avoid processed foods high in refined sugars and unhealthy fats. Experiment with balanced meals that

include a variety of nutrient-rich ingredients to fuel your body and mind throughout the day.

Proverbial Wisdom:
"You are what you eat." By nourishing our bodies with nutrient-dense foods, we fuel our potential and empower ourselves to live life to the fullest, with vitality, energy, and resilience.

The chemistry of nutrition is a powerful force that shapes our health and vitality. By choosing nutrient-dense foods that fuel our bodies and support optimal function, we can nourish ourselves from the inside out and unlock our full potential for health and well-being. So, embrace the power of food as medicine, knowing that with each bite, you are fueling your body and enriching your life.

## Chapter 14: Balancing Taste, Fuel, and Enjoyment

*Proverbial Insight:*
"Eat well, live well." As we explore the delicate balance of taste, fuel, and enjoyment in our relationship with food, let's uncover how finding harmony between these elements can enhance our well-being and enrich our lives.

Food is not only about sustenance; it's also about pleasure and enjoyment. In this chapter, we'll delve into the art of balancing taste, fuel, and enjoyment in our diet and discover how finding this equilibrium can lead to a sustainable and fulfilling relationship with food.

Honoring the Pleasure of Taste:
Taste is an integral part of our dining experience, bringing joy and satisfaction to our meals. By

savoring the flavors and textures of our food, we can cultivate a deeper appreciation for the culinary delights that nourish both our bodies and souls.

Practical Application:
Experiment with different flavors and cuisines to discover what tantalizes your taste buds. Try incorporating herbs, spices, and seasonings into your cooking to add depth and complexity to your meals. Remember that enjoying the taste of your food is an essential aspect of a balanced diet.

Fueling Your Body Wisely:
While taste is important, so too is fueling our bodies with the nutrients they need to function optimally. By prioritizing nutrient-dense foods that provide sustained energy and support overall health, we can ensure

that our dietary choices nourish us from the inside out.

Practical Application:
Focus on incorporating a variety of whole foods into your diet, including fruits, vegetables, lean proteins, whole grains, and healthy fats. These foods provide essential nutrients and energy to fuel your body and support overall well-being. Remember that fueling your body wisely is an act of self-care and empowerment.

Finding Enjoyment in Eating:
Eating should be a pleasurable and enjoyable experience, free from guilt or restriction. By approaching food with mindfulness and intention, we can savor each bite and cultivate a positive relationship with eating that promotes overall well-being.

Practical Application:
Practice mindful eating by slowing down and paying attention to your

food as you eat. Notice the flavors, textures, and sensations of each bite, and savor the experience of nourishing your body. Remember that finding enjoyment in eating is a fundamental aspect of living a balanced and fulfilling life.

Proverbial Wisdom:
"Balance is the key to a happy life." By finding harmony between taste, fuel, and enjoyment in our relationship with food, we can nourish our bodies and souls and live with vitality and joy.

Balancing taste, fuel, and enjoyment in our diet is essential for maintaining a healthy and sustainable relationship with food. By honoring the pleasure of taste, fueling our bodies wisely, and finding enjoyment in eating, we can cultivate a balanced approach to nutrition that promotes overall well-being and enriches our lives. So, embrace the art of balancing taste, fuel, and enjoyment in your diet, knowing that with each mindful bite, you are nourishing your body and nurturing your soul.

Summary:
"Empower Your Essence" is not just a book; it's a roadmap to holistic living and vitality. Through exploring nutrition, movement, mindfulness, and more, readers will discover the power within them to nourish their mind, body, and soul. From understanding the chemistry of nutrition to mastering strength and mobility, each chapter offers practical insights and empowering practices for everyday life. By embracing the wisdom shared in these pages, readers will unlock their full potential and embark on a journey of transformation and empowerment. So, let this book be

your guide as you embark on the
path to holistic well-being, knowing
that with each step, you are
empowering your essence and living
a life filled with health, vitality, and
joy.